Distribution, publication, and copying in any form are prohibited and subject to damages.

# TEN HYPNOSES

Copying, publishing, and sharing with third parties are only permitted with the written consent of the author. Please observe the notes on copyright and usage.

Distribution, publication, and copying in any form are prohibited and subject to damages.

Copying, publishing, and sharing with third parties are only permitted with the written consent of the author. Please observe the notes on copyright and usage.

Distribution, publication, and copying in any form are prohibited and subject to damages.

Ingo Michael Simon

# TEN HYPNOSES

## 46
### FALLING ASLEEP AND STAYING ASLEEP

Copying, publishing, and sharing with third parties are only permitted with the written consent of the author. Please observe the notes on copyright and usage.

Distribution, publication, and copying in any form are prohibited and subject to damages.

© 2024 Ingo Michael Simon
All rights reserved.
Independently published
www.ingosimon.com


Important Notes for Urgent Attention:

The contents of this book are based on the practical experiences of the author with hypnosis applications and psychotherapy in a trance state. Although the author has strived for the utmost care, errors or misunderstandings in the presentation cannot be completely excluded. Therapeutic work with people and the application of hypnosis are solely the responsibility of the hypnotist. It cannot be ruled out that parts of this book may be misunderstood or that the application of a presented procedure may cause an undesirable reaction in the client. The author also assumes no co-responsibility if work with a client is carried out with reference to the statements in this book.

The Author:

Ingo Michael Simon studied psychology and education and is a hypnotherapist with practices in southwestern Germany and Switzerland. With the help of hypnosis-supported psychotherapy, he primarily treats people with persistent psychological conditions. His practice focuses on anxiety disorders, pathological compulsions, and psychosomatic illnesses. His therapeutic offerings mainly include classical and modern hypnosis applications and the dreamland therapy he developed himself.

Copying, publishing, and sharing with third parties are only permitted with the written consent of the author. Please observe the notes on copyright and usage.

Distribution, publication, and copying in any form are prohibited and subject to damages.

| | |
|---|---:|
| **INTRODUCTION** | **6** |
| **COPYRIGHT AND USAGE** | **8** |
| **HYPNOSIS 1** | **10** |
| **HYPNOSIS 2** | **15** |
| **HYPNOSIS 3** | **20** |
| **HYPNOSIS 4** | **25** |
| **HYPNOSIS 5** | **29** |
| **HYPNOSIS 6** | **34** |
| **HYPNOSIS 7** | **38** |
| **HYPNOSIS 8** | **43** |
| **HYPNOSIS 9** | **49** |
| **HYPNOSIS 10** | **55** |
| **ALL TITLES IN THE SERIES** | **60** |

Copying, publishing, and sharing with third parties are only permitted with the written consent of the author. Please observe the notes on copyright and usage.

Distribution, publication, and copying in any form are prohibited and subject to damages.

# Introduction

The series "Ten Hypnoses" is very well known in Germany, Austria, and Switzerland as a collection of texts for therapeutic work and is used by numerous psychotherapeutic practices, doctors, therapists, coaches, and other helping professionals. I am pleased to now be able to offer these texts in other countries as well.

Most therapists have their own methods for inducing and deepening trance as well as for exiting trance. Therefore, I have focused on the main part of the hypnosis. The texts in this book can be integrated as the main part into any hypnosis process. The texts in this collection use various hypnosis techniques. I will not explain these in detail, as I assume that users have the appropriate training. It is also not necessary to understand the exact structure or functioning of the different parts. The texts can simply be read aloud, and they will have their effect.

Decide for yourself which text best suits your client or patient at any given time. You can also combine passages from different texts. It is not about using all ten hypnoses in sequence. It is a selection of possibilities.

Copying, publishing, and sharing with third parties are only permitted with the written consent of the author. Please observe the notes on copyright and usage.

I want to emphasize that books cannot replace therapy. Psychotherapy or other therapeutic treatments involve much more. A careful diagnosis is the necessary basis for deciding on the use of methods, including whether hypnosis or one of my texts should be used. Even in this case, preparatory discussions, follow-up discussions during the session, and of course, a therapeutic concept for the sequence of sessions and the content approaches are essential parts of therapy. This cannot and should not be achieved with a collection of texts.

In any case, I wish you much success in your work and I am pleased if my text templates can contribute in a small way.

*Ingo Michael Simon*

Distribution, publication, and copying in any form are prohibited and subject to damages.

# Copyright and Usage

Copying, publishing, and sharing with third parties is prohibited and only permitted with the written consent of the author. Please observe the following copyright and usage guidelines.

This work has been carefully crafted and created to the best of the author's knowledge and personal experience. It comprises text templates and application guidelines for professional hypnosis sessions. The author is a licensed psychotherapist with extensive experience in psychotherapy, coaching, and personal training using hypnotic techniques and methods. Nevertheless, the author and the publisher assume no liability for the accuracy of information, instructions, and advice, nor for any typographical errors. The author and publisher accept no responsibility or liability for the application of these texts and recommendations with clients or patients, nor for any potential consequences or unexpected reactions. It is expressly noted that the application of therapeutic and advisory techniques and formulations lies solely and entirely within the responsibility of the practitioner. This also applies to adherence to the

Copying, publishing, and sharing with third parties are only permitted with the written consent of the author. Please observe the notes on copyright and usage.

boundaries of legally regulated medical and therapeutic practices. The fact that a book containing action proposals is freely available for sale does not imply that its application with clients or patients is permitted for everyone.

# Hypnosis 1

You want to be able to sleep, deeply and soundly ... ... It's your goal ... ... it's your biggest goal ... ... To fall asleep quickly at night and sink deeper and deeper into sleep ... ... to dream peacefully in a deep, deep sleep and simply sleep through until the next morning ... ... Good sleep is your goal ... ... and you're focusing entirely on this goal ... ... it's amazing how you're doing this ... ... and maybe it's tiring and exhausting, focusing so much on sleeping ... ... that's good because tiredness is what helps you the most ... ... Today is the day of change ... ... the beginning of good sleep ... ... the beginning of falling asleep quickly ... ... the beginning of sleeping through the night ... ... You can let yourself fall into a deep sleep even now, because your deepest inner self, your subconscious, hears my words even in sleep ... ... So sleep, if you want ... ... Just sleep if you want ... ...

You carry this thought within you, the thought of falling asleep better ... ... letting go of worrying thoughts and then truly falling asleep well and sleeping through the whole night ... ... letting go of whatever hinders your sleep ... ... You've had this goal for a long time, you've had this wish for a long time ... ... but today, there's more ... ... Today, at this very moment, every good wish can become a firm thought ... ... an unshakable belief ... ... so firm and so stable that you can't help but follow this thought ... ... so that your body can't help but follow this thought ... ... this thought that says ... ... I let go of all disturbances during the night and am rewarded with good sleep ... ... This is the thought of the night ... ... the good and truly stable thought of the night ... ... It now finds its way into your deepest self ... ... ... ... I let go of all disturbances during the night and am rewarded with good sleep ... ...

You can now also rely on your body's help ... ... because it feels the fatigue after the day's strain ... ... your body is truly tired at night, and surely you know the feeling of lying in bed with a truly tired body ... ... You've often experienced being unable to fall asleep easily even with this tired body ... ... but from now on, your body helps you at night with such deep tiredness that you automatically fall asleep ... ... Your body pulls you into a deep sleep at night ... ... Your body pulls you into a really, really deep sleep at night ... ... because today you have firmly implanted this thought in yourself … … It's your thought of the good night that tells you … … I let go of all disturbances during the night and am rewarded with good sleep … … and with this, you feel your body's tiredness even more intensely at night and let yourself fall into deep sleep … …

Sometimes, it's thoughts that can keep us awake, but you now have the sleep thought … … your thought of good sleep … … and sometimes, it's also our emotions that can keep us awake … … But when you look closely, it's not the emotions themselves that keep us awake, not anger, not frustration, and not even disappointment … … It's the judgments we place on our emotions that can keep us awake … … But you're letting go of disturbing thoughts at night … … and if you've decided to do so, and you have decided, then you're also letting go of all judgments about your emotions at night … … because self-judgments are disturbing thoughts … … So you let go of self-judgments at night … … during the day you can think about them, but at night you let go of all self-judgments and self-criticism … … and that's why your emotions can just be there … … and you find good sleep in them … …

You're setting yourself up to do something good, to make it even easier for you to let go of disturbing thoughts at night ... ... because it's really possible ... ... worries and problems don't just disappear overnight, but you can still manage to sleep from now on ... ... and during the day, you deal with the challenges and find solutions ... ... As soon as you lie down to really sleep, you breathe deeply and consciously three times, very deeply ... ... and with each breath, you let go of disturbing thoughts, like in a ritual ... ... three times you breathe in deeply and breathe out even more deeply ... ... and for your mind, this is the signal to immediately let go of all disturbing thoughts ... ... and then, each deep exhale brings you into a very deep tiredness ... ... a tiredness that forces you to sleep ... ... so tired that you can't help but fall asleep and sleep deeply and soundly ... ... Deliberate breathing out, as soon as you lie down to sleep, brings you into such an intense tiredness that you fall asleep ... ... that you really fall asleep and sleep through until morning ... ... Tonight, you'll feel the tiredness ... ... experience how tired you are and how well you can fall asleep ... ...

Good sleep is waiting for you ... ... good sleep is waiting for you at home, in your bed ... ... you've experienced a great change within yourself, you've set it up yourself ... ... You have firmly implanted a good and helpful thought in your subconscious ... ... your thought of good sleep ... ... your thought that says ... ... I let go of all disturbances during the night and am rewarded with good sleep ... ... and because you are now so deeply relaxed, in a truly special trance, this thought also becomes the truth of your body ... ... Maybe you're wondering what's special about this trance ... ... or you simply feel it inside, sensing that this trance is truly special ... ... Your good sleep will prove it to you ... ... Your good sleep will show you that this trance was different ... ... and your sleep will also be different ... ... Good sleep is waiting for you ... ...

# Hypnosis 2

You have the goal of doing something for a good and deep sleep right now … … to take action and help your body fall asleep better at night … … You're holding this goal firmly in your inner focus and concentrating on it … … and that's why you're successful today in ensuring a good night's sleep … … You're successful today because you're focusing so strongly on your goal of good sleep, so strongly … … Your focus is stronger than ever before, you want it today more than ever, you're preparing yourself with all your strength and willpower to truly find the path to good and restful sleep today … … Today you're taking the decisive step … … today you're taking a more important and bigger step than before, and today you're helping yourself to get a good night's sleep … … Today, it's even the case that you're taking the most important step in a long time because today you're choosing a completely different approach than before … … You're successful today … … You're very successful today, more than you thought or expected … … Today you're achieving your goal of good sleep … … already today … …

First, you let your own strength come into your consciousness … … you remember that your strength has already helped you through many challenges in life … … Your strength has often helped you to persevere and stick with it in difficult situations, to keep going and find success in the end … … You can do that today as well … … You're stronger than you think, and you can now consciously feel your own strength … … You can feel it clearly when you concentrate on your feelings … … You're really strong inside, you have this mental ability to find new ways … … and today, you can use your inner strength better than ever before, use it more to your advantage than ever before … … today, you find your best ally in your mental strength … … because with it, you can achieve adjusting yourself internally … … causing your body and your entire organism to fall asleep more easily at night and experience restful sleep … …

Deep inside, you're now finding real peace, and this peace helps you because inner peace makes your body tired and leads you to sleep … … Worrying thoughts can keep you awake, and letting go of thoughts helps with falling asleep … … and now you're preparing to let go of your thoughts … … Now you're preparing deep inside to let go of all thoughts at night, to be free for the night and for good and restful sleep … … and the thoughts are allowed to return only the next day … … Now you're preparing with all your strength and as if it were the most natural thing in the world to let go of absolutely all thoughts at night and to clear your mind … … and then to fall asleep deeply and really restfully … … with gentle dreams and a peaceful feeling … … All worry thoughts can now go away … … they can go now and make you tired … … All worry thoughts are now actually being released from your inner self, detaching and moving away … … and you're coming to more peace than you thought … … much more peace than you thought … … Now all worry thoughts really must go, they're now leaving you … … now you're really letting go, letting go of all worries … … and now you're feeling the tiredness that comes with it … … tiredness that accompanies you into sleep … …

And deep inside you, positive thoughts and memories are awakening … … Positive thoughts are taking the place of daytime worries … … Now positive and constructive thoughts are awakening within you … … Now you're diving into a beautiful memory … … a very beautiful memory … … this beautiful memory now accompanies you in your tiredness and it accompanies you at night in your tiredness … … This beautiful memory accompanies you every night into sleep … … into truly restful sleep … … It's the most beautiful memory you have … … or the most beautiful fantasy you can imagine … … and this most beautiful memory now also accompanies you into the most beautiful tiredness … … and every night, this most beautiful memory accompanies you in your tiredness and makes you even more tired … … Every night, this most beautiful memory accompanies you into the most beautiful sleep … … every night into the most beautiful sleep … …

With these words, everything inside you changes because you're actually succeeding in sleeping better at night … … because all the words you hear are deeply anchored in your inner self and become your truth … … You're doing a wonderful job of sleeping better at night … … tonight you'll already feel the effect, because tonight you'll fall asleep more easily than before … … Tonight you'll sleep deeper than before … … Tonight you're achieving much more than ever before because today you're truly establishing your good and restful night's sleep … … You've done well and you're still doing well … … it's truly amazing how well you're succeeding today in making good sleep a reality and already experiencing it tonight … … You can be proud of yourself and thank yourself for it … … you can praise yourself because you're the one who has changed everything … … It's only my words, but you're making them true … … You … …

So, good, the most important step has been taken … … Good sleep has now become possible … … and what's possible will also happen … … You're successful … … Good and restful sleep is already coming to you tonight … … like a gift from you to yourself … … a good gift from you to yourself … … Better sleep than you had hoped for is spreading within you tonight, giving you a truly restful night … … already tonight … … and from night to night, your sleep will become deeper and more restful … … deeper and more restful … … until you've achieved the optimal sleep for you … … truly restful sleep that makes you completely satisfied … …

# Hypnosis 3

You have a clear goal … … You want to be able to fall asleep quickly at night … … fall asleep quickly and peacefully and then sleep through the whole night … … You want to let go of everything disturbing and want to sleep restfully … … and that's exactly what's actually possible … … it's possible to find the path of good sleep … … and it's also possible to walk the path of good sleep … … You're walking it today … … yes, you're walking the path of good sleep today … … today you're learning how it's done … … today you're teaching your body how to fall asleep well and sleep restfully … … even to sleep through, just as you want … … Your body can do this … … Your body is preparing today to experience good sleep every night … … Your entire organism is preparing today to experience good sleep every night … … today, you're succeeding more than ever before … … today, you're succeeding particularly well … … particularly well … …

Now, pay attention to your body, feel along your body, and feel the calm and relaxation of your body … … also feel the tiredness and heaviness of your body … … maybe your body also feels lighter in tiredness ... ... Feel how your body feels now because this is the feeling of tiredness that shows itself in it ... ... When we come to rest, become really tired and increasingly tired, our body becomes sluggish and slow ... ... our body shows us that it wants to sleep ... ... your body is showing you this feeling now ... ... Perceive it ... ... Now perceive the feeling of tiredness in your body ... ... Feel your body parts and check which part has already become the most tired ... ...

... ... Feel your head and check how tired it has already become ... ... maybe very tired ... ... so tired that you want to sleep ... ... Then feel your shoulders and check how they feel ... ... how much tiredness can already be felt in your shoulders ... ... and even with the tiredness of the shoulders, your body is asking for rest and for sleep ... ... but maybe there are body parts that are even more tired and demand sleep even more than the shoulders ... ... maybe your arms ... ... Your arms are resting quietly next to your body, and in them, too, you can feel that there is a need for rest and for sleep ... ... your arms are also getting more tired and want to sleep ... ... Both arms feel this tiredness and you perceive that ... ... You perceive that your arms want to sleep ... ...

and also your hands ... ... Feel into your hands and find out how they feel ... ... how much physical tiredness can already be felt in your hands ... ... because your hands also want to rest ... ... your hands are longing for sleep ... ... both hands want to sleep ... ...

... ... Then you feel your upper body ... ... feel what it feels ... ... tiredness ... ... and with each breath, the tiredness becomes stronger and clearer ... ... you're becoming increasingly tired with each breath ... ... so tired that you really want to sleep ... ... Maybe your upper body is the most tired part of your body ... ... or maybe your legs are even more tired ... ... perhaps your legs are so tired that they don't want to move at all ... ... that they want to sleep ... ... Your legs want to sleep ... ... sleep deeply ... ... And finally, you also perceive your feet ... ... your feet, which may now rest more than any other part of your body because they do the most work during the day ... ... they carry you all day and need the most rest at night ... ... and maybe your feet are the most tired ... ... That could be, but it could also be different ... ...

... ... Go through your entire body once more ... ... like a scanner that scans your body and now finds the most tired part … … or the most tired spot … … maybe an arm or a leg … … or the head, which has become tired inside … … the head, which now no longer wants to think but only to feel … … You find the most tired spot of your body or the most tired part … … Now … … and you focus entirely on this spot, on this body part … … to feel the tiredness even more … … to feel the tiredness completely now … … and from there, the tiredness spreads throughout your whole body, making you entirely tired … … from there, the need to sleep spreads throughout your entire body … … Your whole body is just as tired as the most tired spot you've found … … and it becomes even more tired and more tired … … and you feel the strong urge to finally fall asleep … … because now the tiredness is spreading evenly throughout your entire body … … enveloping you completely … … and your organism is learning at this moment how to be completely tired … … and to experience tiredness throughout your entire body … … also and especially in your thoughts, which are becoming tired … … In the past, your body was tired, but your thoughts kept you awake … … now you're changing that … … Now you're making sure that your tiredness envelops your entire body … … now you're making sure that your tiredness envelops your entire organism … … now you're making sure that your tiredness envelops and floods your thoughts, too … … and with that, you're becoming so tired that you let go of your thoughts and really fall asleep … … you can fall asleep deeply … … Now … …

Now enjoy the peace and relaxation … … enjoy the relaxation of your body and your thoughts … … and trust that from now on, you'll also enjoy the relaxation and peace of your body at night, in sleep … … in deep sleep … … trust that from now on, you'll also enjoy the relaxation and peace of your thoughts at night, in sleep … … in deep sleep … … because that's now possible … … Deep sleep is finally possible because your tiredness spreads evenly and intensely throughout your entire body every night … … your tiredness spreads evenly and intensely throughout your entire organism every night … … And every evening, when you lie down and want to sleep, your body remembers to become very tired and to sleep … … Every evening, your deepest inner self remembers to become truly very tired and to fall deeply asleep … … to fall deeply asleep … …

# Hypnosis 4

You want to finally be able to sleep well ... ... You want to find rest at night and recuperation in peaceful sleep ... ... and this goal has brought you here ... ... to finally achieve what you want to achieve and what you can achieve ... ... just falling asleep ... ... and then finding deep rest in sleep ... ... such deep rest that you can sleep through the whole night and only wake up in the morning when the alarm wakes you or when you want to wake up ... ... Today, you're succeeding because today you can approach your goal differently ... ... differently than before ... ... calmer and yet more effectively ... ... calmly and relaxed, achieving the goal of good sleep ... ... You're fully aligning yourself internally with achieving your goal of good sleep ... ... Now ... ...

Imagine you're lying in a very comfortable hammock ... ... outside, in nature ... ... perhaps in a beautiful garden, and it's warm and pleasant ... ... The sun is shining, and you feel good ... ... You feel the warmth of the sun and make yourself really comfortable in your hammock ... ... so comfortable that you'd like to sleep ... ... and you're tired ... ... So you decide to fall asleep in this comfortable position you're in now and experience a restful sleep … … You look up, gazing at the sky … … Your eyes are already closing because you're getting more and more tired … … more and more tired … … You watch the white clouds in the sky, observing how they slowly move in the gentle wind … … and your eyes keep closing because you're so tired and want to sleep … … The sight of the white clouds also lets your thoughts drift away … … your thoughts are like clouds in the sky, slowly drifting away … … far away and insignificant … …

The wind slowly drives the white clouds apart in the sky … … they slowly and leisurely drift away, and more and more, the clear sky behind them becomes visible … … and between the clouds, you see letters in the sky … … There's a sentence there, and you wait until the clouds reveal it … … Meanwhile, you're getting more and more tired … … wanting to sleep, that's how tired you're getting … … and as you fall asleep, you can see the sentence that flows deep into your thoughts … … up there, it says … …

I entrust all my worries to my inner wisdom and rejoice in restful sleep until morning.

... [Read the affirmation slowly and a bit louder than the previous text to emphasize it slightly. Then pause for about 30 seconds before continuing.] ...

And as you fall asleep, this sentence flows deeply into your innermost self ... ... and the words of the sky work deeply and intensely ... ... and you fall asleep ... ... you're so tired that you fall into a deep sleep ... ... and indeed all your worrying thoughts and burdens go to your inner wisdom ... ... to a deep part that takes care of everything while you sleep deeply and soundly ... ... and this sentence from the sky ... ... this belief, this affirmation, ingrains itself deeply within you ... ... so deeply that the affirmation you heard and read in the sky becomes your deep conviction ... ... a deep truth that you can strengthen again and again ... ... that you can repeat internally again and again ... ... and a part of you silently and quietly repeats this beautiful and helpful belief for you ... ... to give you even more peace and to really help you sleep well at night ... ... It's your thought of restful sleep ... ... your thought of restful sleep ... ...

Deep inside, these words are ingrained in you, the words you heard and read in the sky and can look at again and take in once more ... ...

I entrust all my worries to my inner wisdom and rejoice in restful sleep until morning.

… [Read the affirmation slowly and a bit louder than the previous text to emphasize it slightly. Then pause for about 30 seconds before continuing.] …

… … Well done, the words are taking effect and giving you good and restful sleep … … every night … … restful sleep every night … … because this new belief is so deeply anchored within you that it has to work … … that it has to work for you every day … … and give you good and restful sleep … … give you restful sleep every day … …

Your belief helps you tonight and every night … … and every day, you can repeat it, make it more stable … … and especially in the evening, when you want to sleep, you can think it or say it again consciously, because every repetition helps you to really sleep well and to really sleep through … … to find rest … … and good sleep … … truly good sleep … …

# Hypnosis 5

You want to sleep better at night … … You've experienced how it is to have difficulty falling asleep … … and not being able to sleep through the night properly … … that's why you're here today … … to take action … … to experience a deep change within yourself … … a real change that helps you fall asleep well … … really well and quickly fall asleep … … and then sleep through the whole night … … In the state of trance, as comfortable and calm as you are right now, it's possible to find help from your subconscious … … more help than in a waking state, where you have the same goal but perhaps also more reservations and skepticism … … Now you can speak to your subconscious yourself and decide what should be … … how you need to fall asleep and sleep through … … Your subconscious helps you because it hears and understands my words, which become yours … … So it's also you yourself who says … …

… … I can fall asleep and sleep through well … … because I understand that I can also accept and solve all worries and problems during the day … …

… … I can fall asleep and sleep through well … … because I understand that I find the strength for all challenges in deep sleep … …

… … I can fall asleep and sleep through well … … because I understand that deep within, while I sleep, I find new solutions for the day … …

… … I can fall asleep and sleep through well … … because I understand that this helps me stay capable and much better able to master all challenges … …

… … I can do it … … I can really do it … …

… … My active thoughts focus on the day, and at night, when I want to sleep, I let go of all thoughts … … because only then do I become very tired and fall asleep immediately … …

… … My active thoughts focus on the day, and at night, when I want to sleep, I let go of all thoughts … … because letting go of thoughts helps me fall into a deep sleep … …

… … My active thoughts focus on the day, and at night, when I want to sleep, I let go of all thoughts … … because that's how I fall into deep sleep and deep dreams … …

… … My active thoughts focus on the day, and at night, when I want to sleep, I let go of all thoughts … … because then I succeed in falling asleep and sleeping through … …

… … I can do it … … I can really do it … …

… … My body supports me every night in sleeping with relaxation and tiredness … … and that's why I can really fall asleep very well … …

… … My body supports me every night in sleeping with relaxation and tiredness … … and that's why I already relax when I lie down in bed … …

… … My body supports me every night in sleeping with relaxation and tiredness … … and that's why my sleep is restful and refreshing … …

… … My body supports me every night in sleeping with relaxation and tiredness … … and that's why I can fall asleep well, dream peacefully, and really sleep through … …

… … I can do it … … I can really do it … …

… … I allow my feelings and accept them … … because I've understood that this is how I become calmer and find true inner peace … …

… … I allow my feelings and accept them … … because I've understood that this is how my thoughts become calmer and I can sleep better … …

… … I allow my feelings and accept them … … because I've understood that without judgments and without self-criticism, I come to rest much better and more quickly … …

… … I allow my feelings and accept them … … because I've understood that this makes it much easier for me to fall asleep, that it makes it much easier for me to sleep through … …

… … I can do it … … I can really do it … …

… … I now fall asleep peacefully at night and sleep through the whole night … … and that's why I can take much more and better care of myself during the day … …

… … I now fall asleep peacefully at night and sleep through the whole night … … and that's why I praise myself and pat myself on the back … …

… … I now fall asleep peacefully at night and sleep through the whole night … … and that's why I'm already looking forward to the coming night … …

… … I now fall asleep peacefully at night and sleep through the whole night … … and that's why I give myself more recognition and respect … …

… … I do it … … I really do it … … [Now pause for about 30 seconds] … …

Well done … … You've understood it deeply within … … Let all the words you've heard take effect and trust that they are your own and will come true just as you've heard them … … All words flow deeply into your subconscious … … and develop there for your best … … so that you can really sleep well … … already sleep better today than before … … and with each day, your sleep will get better and better … … until you feel completely satisfied … … You can do it … … You can really do it … …

# Hypnosis 6

You want to finally be able to sleep properly again ... ... to sleep restfully ... ... You know that it was heavy thoughts and worries that kept you awake ... ... sometimes even worries that you didn't really perceive ... ... but somehow there were still thoughts of sorrow and worry within you ... ... or fears that kept you awake ... ... But whatever exactly could keep you awake can also find its solutions during the day ... ... it's possible to sleep at night, especially in difficult times because that's when you need restful sleep even more ... ... You're now ready to accept and sort out what could rob you of sleep, to sleep well from now on ... ... So you're turning to an entity that can help you ... ... an entity you can believe in because it can really help you ... ... and my words become your thoughts ... ... my words become your words, which you speak within yourself along with me ... ... You say ... ...

Dear Subconscious / Dear Inner Helper / Dear Guardian Angel ... ... I ask for support in moving the obstacles of the night to the day because I know that I can solve problems and worries much better during the day than at night ... ... I ask for support in finally finding peace at night and sleeping so well that I can truly recover ... ... with all my strength, I want to let go of the obstacles of the night, and you can help me with that ... ... Give me support in really letting go at night, especially letting go of what I don't perceive as a disturbance or obstacle, even though it hinders my sleep ... ... Dear Subconscious / Dear Inner Helper / Dear Guardian Angel ... ... together with you, I can do this ... ...

Dear Subconscious / Dear Inner Helper / Dear Guardian Angel ... ... support me in feeling my body's tiredness at night and with all my mindfulness, allow it ... ... so that I can also accept this tiredness with my thoughts and fully embrace it, to become tired ... ... to feel tiredness and sleep throughout my entire body and mind at night and to fully follow this feeling ... ... Dear Subconscious / Dear Inner Helper / Dear Guardian Angel ... ... support me in falling asleep quickly and in processing the day constructively in my dreams ... ... then I can definitely succeed in processing my feelings constructively and calmly in my dreams, so that the whole night is marked by peaceful sleep ... ...

Dear Subconscious / Dear Inner Helper / Dear Guardian Angel ... ... I know that I need to take better care of myself

… … that I also need to pay attention to myself and my feelings during the day … … and to only carry the responsibility that truly belongs to me … … I can also reduce burdens that don't belong to me … … Please support me in recognizing when I need rest and balance … … and that I recognize in time when I'm taking on too much … … that I also recognize in time when I'm taking on responsibility and handling things that I'm not actually responsible for … … Dear Subconscious / Dear Inner Helper / Dear Guardian Angel … … I trust in your support and guidance … … I trust that I will receive help on this path and that I can help myself best … …

Dear Subconscious / Dear Inner Helper / Dear Guardian Angel … … please also support me in meeting myself with patience and mindfulness … … that I can accept myself better and accept that I'm not perfect and don't have to be perfect … … I know it's helpful for me to accept myself … … it's even better if I succeed in loving myself … … even if I don't achieve my goals as quickly or easily as I wish … … Dear Subconscious / Dear Inner Helper / Dear Guardian Angel … … with your support, I can definitely accept and love myself better … … especially if it takes a few more days before I can really sleep well again ... ... that's when I need it the most, to accept and like myself, to be able to love myself ... ... Self-love, I know, is the key to every constructive change ... ... Dear Subconscious / Dear Inner Helper / Dear Guardian Angel ... ... Thank you for your support ... ...

Now, lean back internally and trust that your words will find their way to the entity that can help you and that you'll really receive support ... ... Support from your helper entity, which becomes help within you ... ... because deep within you, there's always a helper entity that was addressed by these words ... ... So your inner self is preparing to do everything necessary to truly enable good sleep ... ... as quickly as possible ... ... as quickly as possible ... ...

# Hypnosis 7

You're here today to find good sleep again ... ... truly good sleep, just like it used to be ... ... You remember a time of good sleep, when sleep was still restful ... ... You know that this time existed, and today it's possible to reactivate the feeling of that time ... ... today it's possible to renew the memory and the path of good sleep ... ... and with that, let your sleep become good again from now on, just as it was before when you could sleep so well ... ... so that you can already sleep better today ... ... so that you can lie down relaxed for the night and really find sleep quickly and easily ... ... restful sleep ... ... You're now preparing for this ... ... Today you're succeeding in reactivating this good sleep from the past because you're ready for it ... ... You're truly ready for it now ... ...

In your feelings, you're taking a journey through space and time ... ... to go back to a time in your life when you could still sleep really well ... ... You're crossing images and memories on your journey ... ... encountering feelings and thoughts you had before ... ... maybe certain situations in your life come to mind immediately on this journey, and it's as if you're taking a quick flight over your life … … with a view of everything that has happened … … and if you want, you can focus on the events or simply look past them and just take this journey to soon arrive in a time before the sleeplessness … … to be in a time before the sleepless nights … … to arrive in a time of continuous sleep because that time existed … … You could sleep better in the past, maybe not always … … there were times when you could sleep very well … … others when you could sleep less well, but then you managed to return to good sleep … … and on your journey, you're getting closer to this time now … … It's as if you're making a big leap into a time of good sleep, to feel it once again … … For this, you don't have to achieve anything, don't have to do anything great or come up with a trick … … no need to have a clear memory with images … … Just imagine that you're arriving at the time when you could sleep well … … In your feelings, you can bridge many years in just a single moment and go very far back, if you want … …

Now, pay attention to your feelings … … to your mood and also to the feeling of your body … … because now the feeling of good sleep is within you ... ... as a memory of your life, because no memory is ever lost ... ... you could just sleep well at night, you took care of your worries during the day ... ... maybe you didn't even have any real worries and could therefore sleep so well ... ... In the past, this was completely normal for you, it was just the way it was, you could sleep ... ... and this memory is still within you ... ... it's also stored in your body because the body stores every feeling ... ... Feel where you are ... ... in which time of your life you could still sleep so well ... ... Consider how old you were when you could sleep so well ... ... Also consider in what environment you are, where your journey has taken you ... ... and then dive deep into these images or simply into the feeling of the time ... ... into the feeling of good sleep ... ... of easy falling asleep and deep sleeping ... ... into the feeling of sleeping through ... ... into the feeling of a peaceful night ... ... a truly peaceful and completely restful night ... ... You're in your thoughts back in this time ... ... and this feeling of sleep, this path of good sleep, is being reactivated within you ... ... because now your body remembers how it was ... ... now your entire organism remembers how it's done, really sleeping well ... ... You remember deep inside how it's done, especially in difficult times and with problems, to fall asleep well and use sleep to recharge ... ... You remember ... ...

Your subconscious lets this inner program of good sleep come alive again ... ... because now it's really possible ... ... your old program of good sleep becomes your new sleep program ... ... your inner self holds on to the good sleep ... ... and with this good sleep program, you continue your journey ... ... It takes you into the future ... ... You go with the ability of good sleep from the past directly into the future ... ... and your good sleep program is active again ... ... good sleep is available to you again ... ... with the good sleep, you go from the present into the future ... ... Now ... ... Now ... ... into a future with good sleep because you're using your sleep program from back then ... ... Now ... ... Now ... ... You now look at pictures of the future ... ... You imagine and see before your inner eye what it will be like ... ... You see that you can sleep well again, just as it was normal in the past ... ... It becomes normal again ... ... In your future, in your near future, you'll sleep like a log ... ...

Let the image of good sleep become really clear, really conscious ... ... In the near future, you'll sleep like a log again ... ... and with this idea and with confidence, your journey returns to the present ... ... with good sleep ... ... with the available program of good sleep ... ... and in your present, already in the coming night, your sleep program will help you ... ... Your subconscious gives you the sleep from back then in the coming night ... ... the good sleep from back then, which you'll also have in the future ... ...

# Hypnosis 8

### Instructions for the Procedure

Ideomotoric signals are phenomena where our body follows our feelings and thoughts with movements. In everyday life, this following is shown as body posture, muscle tension, and movement patterns of a person that naturally change with the mood and thoughts. In trance, ideomotoric signals can be used to receive information that the client cannot actively share. The subconscious can, for example, answer questions with an agreed finger signal. Of course, ideomotoric reactions can also be used suggestively, for example, with arm levitations and catalepsies. An ideomotoric approach strengthens trust in hypnosis and in one's ability to change, thus promoting therapy.

**+++ End of Instructions +++**


Today you want to do something to finally be able to sleep well again ... ... to fall asleep well and sleep through the night ... ... and that works best in cooperation with your subconscious ... ... because in trance, in the beautiful deep relaxation you're feeling now, you can really work with your subconscious, and above all, your subconscious can and will confirm and prove to you that it's helping you ... ... Your subconscious will confirm and prove to you that you're successful together and that you'll really sleep better from now on ... ... I'll show you how that works ... ... Maybe you're already quite curious about how it works, that your subconscious gives you a real sign ... ... one that you can recognize and verify ... ... You can experience that today, in just a few minutes ... ... So, let's go ... ...

Changes can always happen when we manage to build and maintain a clear picture of our goal ... ... and this clear picture of the goal can then take effect ... ... imprinting itself so deeply that it becomes the next truth in our life ... ... and you want the truth of good sleep to emerge ... ... So, it's now important to have a clear picture of your goal ... ... a clear picture of your good sleep ... ... You simply have to imagine now how it is when you can sleep the way you want ... ... Imagine that and concentrate intensely on this idea ... ... First, create a picture of how you can lie best ... ... on your back or sideways ... ... or on your stomach ... ... Consider and imagine how you can lie best ... ... Imagine watching yourself sleeping ... ... and stay concentrated on this visual idea ... ... Watch yourself sleeping comfortably before your inner eye ... ... Then create a picture of how you fall asleep ... ... maybe a picture of your eyes slowly closing because you're too tired to keep them open ... ... Your eyes are closing, and you keep them closed because it's much more pleasant ... ... Watch yourself doing this because with this visual idea, with this visualization, your deep inner self is preparing for this good sleep ... ... The picture imprints itself on you and becomes the next truth ... ... Now consider and imagine how you sleep through the whole night ... ... maybe very deeply and soundly ... ... maybe with beautiful dreams in your sleep ... ... Imagine that you're lying in bed and really sleeping and that you actually have beautiful dreams ... ... dreams that deepen your sleep ... ... Imagine a picture where you're lying very calmly and relaxed and sleeping ... ... peacefully and very comfortably ... ... That's how your nights should be and stay ... ... that's exactly how your nights should be and stay ... ...

Stay entirely in this picture ... ... imagine it like a photo or like a still image from a video ... ... and this picture should imprint on your nights … … because that's how you want to sleep, and that's how you can sleep … … Your subconscious helps you with that … … The more you manage to maintain this picture and see it before your inner eye, the better your subconscious can make this picture your next truth … … to truly good night's sleep … … and as soon as your subconscious has accomplished that, and it will accomplish it, your right hand closes into a fist … … as a sign that you can really hold this inner picture and that it becomes your truth … … Your subconscious will show you when it's ready, when it has taken it over for you like that … … The longer you concentrate on the picture of good sleep, the more your right hand closes into a fist … … Step by step, your right hand closes into a fist, and as soon as it's closed, your good sleep has become the new truth in your life … … Your subconscious will do it, it will close your hand and tell you that you'll sleep well … … already tonight and every upcoming night as well as possible … … Your subconscious closes your hand, and above all … … Your subconscious doesn't lie … … It keeps its promise … … Your hand closes into a fist … … and you sleep well … …

[Please try to be patient until the hand closes. Ideomotoric signals are reliable signs, similar to kinesiological muscle tests. Here we're working with a mixture of suggestive prompts and ideomotoric communication. By repeatedly saying ... Your hand closes into a fist ... it has a suggestive effect, and the ideomotoric response occurs. By assuming that good sleep is connected with this, a link is established in the subconscious. At the same time, the subconscious confirms the good sleep. If it couldn't produce good sleep, it wouldn't make sense to close the hand. So, if the closing happens only due to suggestion, it's still proof of the effect for the conscious mind, as that was the agreement. If the conscious mind is convinced, the goal is almost achieved.]

Your subconscious has imprinted the image of good sleep, and that's why you'll really sleep well ... ... Your hand is now becoming fully mobile again, and you can open it ... ... Your subconscious is handing you back full control of your hand, which can feel good ... ... You can check it ... ... Move your hand or both hands and fingers and check that your hands are fully under your conscious control ... ...

[Always make sure that the client has regained full conscious and active control of their hands and fingers and can move them. Let them actively try. If it doesn't work, help with further suggestions ... Your hands and fingers are totally relaxed, completely loose. Your hands and fingers are very, very loose ... You can move them ...]

Your subconscious has created good sleep with you ... ... You helped with your visual idea and your subconscious with the imprinting of the picture and with the feedback of the closed fist as proof that you'll sleep better from now on ... ... Isn't it good that this proof is possible in trance? ... ... Yes, it's good ... ...

# Hypnosis 9

## Instructions for the Procedure

A self-hypnosis trigger is a signal that initiates the state of trance. With its help, even an inexperienced client can continue working with self-hypnosis at home. Of course, they can "only" work with simple suggestions that they can easily remember and that we should prepare, or with simple visualizations. Triggered self-hypnosis is a very good tool to give the client a task to take home and to promote the therapy. This way, the time between sessions in the practice doesn't go without therapy but is continued at home. Completely self-directed self-hypnosis, without a trigger, is also easy to learn but takes a lot of time and practice. Setting up the trigger is a relatively simple task and naturally relieves the client, whom I don't want to burden with the training of a self-directed self-hypnosis. Despite all the naysayers, I also claim here that it's really not a problem to teach a client simple trigger self-hypnosis. It's no more dangerous than meditation or autogenic training or yoga. You can also survive those unscathed at home. I have experienced numerous patients in my practice who not only managed well with self-hypnosis but also enjoyed it. And if a patient enjoys doing self-hypnosis, no matter how simple the suggestion may seem, it's a very good support for compliance. Discuss the procedure once before the hypnosis and give the client a brief, bullet-point list of the steps of self-hypnosis so that they have a little guide.

**+++ End of Instructions +++**


Today you're learning how to do self-hypnosis because with self-hypnosis, you can find good and restful sleep even more quickly … … You can do self-hypnosis just before sleeping, but also during the day as preparation for good night's sleep … … You can do it as often as you like … … each self-hypnosis helps you improve your sleep, increase your sleep quality … … Now, concentrate on your relaxation, on the state of trance you're in now … … This is how trance feels … … calm and relaxed, yet completely normal … … a state that you can create yourself … … It's very simple and completely safe, because I'll show you how it works … … and you'll automatically learn how to enter a pleasant state of trance yourself and do something good for yourself ... ... Feel the relaxation now clearly ... ... Feel how good it feels to be relaxed ... ... in trance and at the same time being able to hear everything ... ... and also being able to think ... ...

You can create this state yourself ... ... you can also go into trance at home ... ... You use a code word for this that's just for you ... ... The code word is ... ... Iamon ... [Please emphasize the made-up word on the I ... I-amon.] ... ... Make yourself comfortable at home and close your eyes, just like here ... ... and then whisper this word over and over again until you notice that it's making you tired ... ... and that happens after just a few repetitions ... ... So, whisper ... ... Iamon – Iamon – Iamon – Iamon – Iamon – Iamon ... ... and in doing so, you automatically go into a pleasant trance ... ... maybe just as deep as here ... ... but it's enough to enter a very light trance ... ... Your code word Iamon will now be deeply anchored in your subconscious, so you can use this word whenever you want to enter trance ... ...

You can then deepen your trance yourself by whispering ten times ... ... I relax and let go ... ... You simply whisper ... ... I relax once and let go ... ... I relax twice and let go ... ... I relax three times and let go ... ... and so on ... ... until you finally reach ten and whisper ... ... I relax ten times and let go ... ... and in doing so, you enter a pleasantly deep state of relaxation ... ... A part of you enters a really nice, deep trance, and another part stays awake and controls your trance ... ... You're completely safe in this ... ...

[For deepening and the main part, I recommend counting with the suggestions ... once ... twice, etc. This has the advantage that the client isn't distracted by wondering how many times they've repeated the suggestion. It doesn't really matter if it's exactly ten repetitions, but in trance, it's easier to keep the thread this way. You can also speak all ten repetitions out loud. After all, you're also working suggestively in this hypnosis. So, it's not just self-hypnosis training but also a hypnosis.]

Then comes the main part, the most important part of your self-hypnosis ... ... and in this part, you work with a beautiful and helpful suggestion ... ... You simply whisper it ten times ... ... Ten times you say ... ... I sleep better tonight than ever before ... ... Again, you count while doing this ... ... You say ... ... I sleep better tonight than ever before, once ... ... I sleep better tonight than ever before, twice ... ... I sleep better tonight than ever before, three times ... ... until you finally say … … I sleep better tonight than ever before, ten times … … and then you simply rest in your pleasant trance for a while … … if you want, and when the time is right, you can fall asleep directly … … or you'll wake up once more and then later go to bed to sleep … …

To wake yourself up again, imagine freezing cold rain … … Imagine standing in freezing cold rain, and then you say … … I want to be awake now … … and then you count energetically to three and open your eyes … … It's very simple … … once again … … To wake yourself up again, imagine standing in freezing cold rain, and then you say … … I want to be awake now – One – Two – Three … … and then you're awake and open your eyes … … It's very simple, and you can try it later … …

You've already learned how it works … … how you can create self-hypnosis and do something to sleep better and better … … Your subconscious has learned for you to go into trance immediately with your code word, and you know what to do next … …

… … Your code word Iamon brings you into trance, which you deepen with the words I relax and let go … … Then follows your suggestion ... I sleep twice as well tonight as before ... and then you imagine freezing cold rain and say ... I want to be awake now – One – Two – Three ... ...

# Hypnosis 10

Close your eyes and allow yourself to rest now and do nothing at all ... ... Let go of all thoughts and dream yourself to a beautiful place ... ... to a place in your imagination that's more beautiful than anything you've ever seen in your waking life ... ... beautiful nature around you and a completely relaxed feeling inside you ... ... You're there with just a single thought ... ... You think this thought now and arrive there ... ... at this special place in your own imagination ... ... Imagination and reality sometimes lie very close together ... ... and sometimes even are one and the same ... ... starting as imagination and in the next moment becoming reality because you want it so ... ... This is the land of dreams ... ... the land of your dreams ... ... Here you can feel your emotions more clearly and view your memories more vividly than in your waking life ... ... You're in the land of dreams ... ...

You're tired and want to sleep ... ... especially since sleeping has been so difficult lately ... ... In the land of dreams, you want to find good sleep ... ... here it's possible because here, everything is possible that you can think of … … You're standing in front of a house … … it's an old house, a mansion that looks grand and ornate … … and above the entrance door hangs a large sign that reads … … Hotel of Good Sleep … … and because you so much want to sleep well again, you enter this hotel to find good sleep there … … You enter the lobby and go to the reception … … There, a friendly lady hands you a key to your room … … In the land of dreams, you can't surprise anyone; everyone here knows you're on your way, and everyone helps you … … You take the key and go to your room … … A friendly staff member of the house accompanies you there … …

… … You enter the room … … It looks like your bedroom … … The same furniture is here … … Your bed is in this room … … and on the bed lies a thick book … … You go to the bed and would love to lie down and sleep … … But first, you take the book in your hand … … On the cover of the book is written … … Book of Good Sleep … … You open the book and flip through it … … but there are only blank pages … … on some of these pages, there are headings, but no text … … It's not about reading in this book … … The Book of Good Sleep has a completely different task, a completely different function ... ... it's the book into which you can write ... ... You look around and discover a pen ... ... It's lying on the bed ... ... You take it in your hand and then make yourself really comfortable on the bed ... ... You lie down and make yourself as comfortable as possible so that you could sleep the best ... ...

... ... Then you flip through the Book of Good Sleep until you find the first heading ... ... there it says ... ... What Makes Me Angry ... ... just this heading, and you think about what makes you most angry at the moment ... ... or what has particularly angered you recently ... ... because anger could keep you awake ... ... and you write your anger in the book ... ... maybe a word or a sentence ... ... or you write a name in it ... ... the name of a person who angers you or who you've been angry with ... ... Then you turn the page and find the next heading ... ... and again, the page is blank so that you can fill it with your thoughts ... ... write your thoughts into the book ... ...

... ... There it says ... ... What Makes Me Furious ... ... just this heading, and you think about what makes you most furious at the moment ... ... or what has particularly made you furious recently ... ... because fury could also keep you awake ... ... fury about injustice, perhaps, or possibly about powerlessness because you can't do anything about certain things ... ... You write your fury in the book ... ... maybe a word or a sentence ... ... or you write a name in it ... ... the name of a person who has something to do with your fury or your powerlessness ... ... that you associate with it ... ... Then you turn the page and find the next heading ... ... and again, the page is blank so that you can fill it with your thoughts ... ... write your thoughts into the book ... ...

... ... The next heading you find is titled ... ... What Has Hurt Me ... ... just this heading, and you think about what has hurt you most recently ... ... or what has hurt you ... ... because hurt and offense could also keep you awake ... ... the feeling of humiliation or the feeling of not being seen ... ... experiencing too little appreciation ... ... You write your hurt in the book ... ... maybe a word or a sentence ... ... or you write a name in it ... ... the name of a person you associate with your hurt and offense ... ... Then you turn the page and find the next heading ... ... and again, the page is blank so that you can fill it with your thoughts ... ... write your thoughts into the book ... ... There it says ... ... What Has Brought Me the Most Joy because there is also joy in your life ... ... and for what has brought you the most joy recently, you write a word or a name in the Book of Good Sleep ... ... Joy helps you fall asleep ... ... Then you become very tired in the land of dreams ... ... You close the book and become more and more tired ... ... so tired that your eyes close ... ... You put the book aside ... ... with your feelings in it ... ... and you lie down, lean back, and fall asleep ... ... You fall deeply and soundly asleep in the land of dreams ... ...

Then you dream the most beautiful dream in a long time ... ... You dream a dream of good sleep and that it always helps you to become aware of your feelings and to express them ... ... just as you wrote them in the Book of Good Sleep in the land of dreams today ... ... You think about how exactly this can also help you in your waking everyday life ... ... the clarity of your feelings and the admission of your feelings ... ... If you can accept and express your feelings, write them deep within you into the Book of Good Sleep, you can sleep well, very well ... ... But where is the Book of Good Sleep? ... ... Where is this book? ... ... In your imagination? ... ... The book is in the land of dreams, and the land of dreams is within you ... ... it has always been there ... ... I'm just telling you about it ... ...

Distribution, publication, and copying in any form are prohibited and subject to damages.

## All Titles in the Series

Volume 1: Smoking Cessation
Volume 2: Anxiety and Restlessness
Volume 3: Burnout
Volume 4: Reducing Overweight
Volume 5: Coping with the Past
Volume 6: Suicidal Thoughts and Attempts
Volume 7: Psycho-Oncology
Volume 8: Obsessions and Tics
Volume 9: Self-Confidence and Decision-Making
Volume 10: Grief Work
Volume 11: Psychosomatics
Volume 12: Chronic Pain
Volume 13: Depressive Thoughts
Volume 14: Panic Attacks
Volume 15: Domestic Violence, Victim Support
Volume 16: Post-Traumatic Stress
Volume 17: Exam Anxiety and Stage Fright
Volume 18: Anti-Violence Training, Offender Support
Volume 19: Addiction Tendencies
Volume 20: Social Phobia and Fear of Contact
Volume 21: Nail Biting
Volume 22: Self-Awareness and Self-Love
Volume 23: Teeth Grinding and Night Clenching
Volume 24: Feelings of Guilt
Volume 25: Fear in Crowds
Volume 26: Fear of Flying, Aviophobia
Volume 27: Fear in Enclosed Spaces, Claustrophobia
Volume 28: Tinnitus, Ear Noises
Volume 29: Fear of Heights
Volume 30: Neurodermatitis

Copying, publishing, and sharing with third parties are only permitted with the written consent of the author. Please observe the notes on copyright and usage.

Volume 31: Finding Inner Balance
Volume 32: Overcoming Loneliness
Volume 33: Fear of Illness, Hypochondria
Volume 34: Anticipatory Anxiety, Fear of Fear
Volume 35: Jealousy in Relationships
Volume 36: Driving Anxiety
Volume 37: New Start after Separation
Volume 38: Fear of Injections
Volume 39: Heart Anxiety Neurosis
Volume 40: Overcoming Resentment and Anger
Volume 41: Resolving Blockages and Positive Thinking
Volume 42: Stress Reduction, Stress Management
Volume 43: Body Relaxation
Volume 44: Deep Relaxation
Volume 45: Fear of the Dark
Volume 46: Falling Asleep and Staying Asleep
Volume 47: Compulsive Buying
Volume 48: Restless Legs Syndrome
Volume 49: Bulimia
Volume 50: Anorexia
Volume 51: Overcoming Nightmares
Volume 52: Imagined Deformity
Volume 53: Overcoming Distrust, Finding Trust
Volume 54: Processing Failures
Volume 55: Humiliation, Emotional Hurt
Volume 56: Distressing Compassion, Vicarious Suffering
Volume 57: Self-Forgiveness
Volume 58: Self-Awareness, Self-Confidence
Volume 59: Saying No
Volume 60: Assertiveness
Volume 61: Setting Boundaries and Self-Assertion
Volume 62: Decision-Making Ability

Volume 63: Success Orientation
Volume 64: Ruminating, Circular Thinking
Volume 65: Accepting Pregnancy
Volume 66: Birth Preparation
Volume 67: Spiritual Opening
Volume 68: Joy of Life and Inner Lightness
Volume 69: Patience and Inner Peace
Volume 70: Fibromyalgia and Rheumatism
Volume 71: Irritable Bowel Syndrome, Crohn's Disease
Volume 72: Fear of Nausea, Emetophobia
Volume 73: Stuttering and Cluttering, Speech Flow Disorders
Volume 74: Concentration and Knowledge Anchoring
Volume 75: Vitality and Spontaneity
Volume 76: Searching for Meaning and Finding Goals
Volume 77: Life Crises, Life Events
Volume 78: Workaholism, Goal Obsession
Volume 79: Helper Syndrome, Helpless Helpers
Volume 80: Medication Abuse
Volume 81: Gambling Addiction
Volume 82: Internet Addiction, Smartphone Addiction
Volume 83: Hoarding Disorder, Compulsive Collecting
Volume 84: Conspiracy Thoughts, Overvalued Ideas
Volume 85: Fear of Operations and Treatments
Volume 86: Fear of Aging
Volume 87: Travel Anxiety
Volume 88: Anxiety When Urinating, Paruresis
Volume 89: Fear of Intimacy and Togetherness
Volume 90: Fear of Blushing
Volume 91: Coming Out in Homosexuality
Volume 92: Charisma Training
Volume 93: Migraines and Chronic Headaches
Volume 94: Overcoming Allergies, Bronchial Asthma

Volume 95: Normalizing Blood Pressure
Volume 96: Compulsive Perfectionism
Volume 97: Sports Hypnosis, Motivation
Volume 98: Sports Hypnosis, Performance Enhancement
Volume 99: Determination and Focus
Volume 100: Encountering the Inner Child
Volume 101: Cravings, Binge Eating
Volume 102: Stimulating Metabolism
Volume 103: Bipolar Mood Swings
Volume 104: Borderline, Identity Crises
Volume 105: Hypomania, Euphoria, Mania
Volume 106: Restlessness, Agitation
Volume 107: Nervous Breakdown
Volume 108: Adjustment Disorders
Volume 109: Self-Alienation, Depersonalization
Volume 110: Ending Self-Pity
Volume 111: Primary Gain of Illness
Volume 112: Secondary Gain of Illness
Volume 113: Bullying, Victim Support
Volume 114: Letting Go of Envy and Jealousy
Volume 115: Fear of Spiders, Arachnophobia
Volume 116: Fear of Dogs or Cats
Volume 117: Fear of Strangers, Xenophobia
Volume 118: Excessive Worries, Generalized Anxiety
Volume 119: Strengthening Sense of Responsibility
Volume 120: Unrequited Love, Heartache
Volume 121: Work-Life Balance
Volume 122: Letting Go of Unattainable Goals
Volume 123: Allowing and Accepting Help
Volume 124: Letting Go of Adult Children
Volume 125: Tourette Syndrome
Volume 126: Life Changes and New Starts

Volume 127: Accepting Life in a Wheelchair
Volume 128: Understanding and Overcoming Homesickness
Volume 129: Understanding and Overcoming Wanderlust
Volume 130: Dizziness, Meniere's Disease
Volume 131: Overcoming Aggression
Volume 132: Cutting and Self-Harm
Volume 133: Hair Pulling, Trichotillomania
Volume 134: Postpartum Depression
Volume 135: For Relatives of Dementia Patients
Volume 136: Self-Harm, Artificial Disorders
Volume 137: Activating Self-Healing Powers
Volume 138: Preventing Depression Relapse
Volume 139: Reactive Psychoses, Follow-Up
Volume 140: Obsessive Thoughts and Impulses
Volume 141: Compulsive Checking
Volume 142: Compulsive Counting, Symmetry Obsession
Volume 143: Compulsive Washing, Cleanliness Obsession
Volume 144: Compulsive Questioning
Volume 145: Dissociative Paralysis
Volume 146: Phantom Pain
Volume 147: Overcoming Complaining
Volume 148: Hay Fever, Pollen Allergy
Volume 149: Sexual Abuse, Victim Support
Volume 150: Standing Strong Against Sexism, #metoo
Volume 151: Binge Eating
Volume 152: Overcoming Thoughts of Revenge
Volume 153: Detachment from the Aggressor, Stockholm Syndrome
Volume 154: Courage to Separate
Volume 155: Chronic Fatigue, Exhaustion
Volume 156: Fear of the Future, Existential Anxiety
Volume 157: Excessive Worry About Children
Volume 158: Fear of Failure

Volume 159: Ending Distrust and Control
Volume 160: Dejection, Dysphoria
Volume 161: Boreout, Chronic Boredom
Volume 162: Bipolar Disorders, Relapse Prevention
Volume 163: Mania, Relapse Prevention
Volume 164: Nihilism, Feelings of Worthlessness
Volume 165: Thumb Sucking
Volume 166: Being Brave
Volume 167: Being Proud
Volume 168: Overcoming Shyness
Volume 169: Being Able to Delegate Responsibility
Volume 170: Being Able to Show Emotions
Volume 171: Letting Go of Guilt, Victim Support
Volume 172: Processing Guilt, Offender Support
Volume 173: Mood Swings, Cyclothymia
Volume 174: Lack of Drive, Vital Sadness
Volume 175: Hearing Voices with Reality Reference
Volume 176: Confident Communication
Volume 177: Standing Up for Oneself
Volume 178: Taking New Paths
Volume 179: Confident Job Application
Volume 180: No Longer Being Taken Advantage Of
Volume 181: End of Submissiveness
Volume 182: Depressive Numbness
Volume 183: Mood Drops, Affective Incontinence
Volume 184: Mood Instability
Volume 185: Somatoform Disorders
Volume 186: Stomach Ulcer, Psychosomatic
Volume 187: Accepting Amputation
Volume 188: Overcoming and Letting Go of Hatred
Volume 189: Ending Accusations
Volume 190: Allowing Tears, Being Able to Cry

Volume 191: Finding and Sorting Repressed Feelings
Volume 192: Somatoform Pain
Volume 193: Living Autonomously
Volume 194: Anhedonia, Joylessness
Volume 195: Persistent Sadness
Volume 196: Obesity, Food Addiction
Volume 197: Parents of Abused Children
Volume 198: Letting Go and Letting Be
Volume 199: Childhood Sexual Abuse
Volume 200: Fear of Loss

www.ingramcontent.com/pod-product-compliance
Lightning Source LLC
Chambersburg PA
CBHW030503220526
45464CB00006B/2634